HOW TO INTERVIEW THE COACH

IT'S NOT WHAT YOU SAY, IT'S WHAT THEY HEAR THAT MATTERS.

KENNETH PARADY

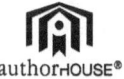

AuthorHouse™
1663 Liberty Drive
Bloomington, IN 47403
www.authorhouse.com
Phone: 1 (800) 839-8640

© 2015 Kenneth Parady. All rights reserved.

No part of this book may be reproduced, stored in a retrieval system, or transmitted by any means without the written permission of the author.

Published by AuthorHouse 01/21/2015

ISBN: 978-1-4969-6477-9 (sc)
ISBN: 978-1-4969-6474-8 (e)

Any people depicted in stock imagery provided by Thinkstock are models, and such images are being used for illustrative purposes only.
Certain stock imagery © Thinkstock.

This book is printed on acid-free paper.

Because of the dynamic nature of the Internet, any web addresses or links contained in this book may have changed since publication and may no longer be valid. The views expressed in this work are solely those of the author and do not necessarily reflect the views of the publisher, and the publisher hereby disclaims any responsibility for them.

To Joyce,

who has given me confidence & support in all I have done the past twenty years. I thank you."

How to Interview the Coach!

National Sports Marketing Group

Developers of the Mental Game Plan

Foreword

As you read this manual, you should already have filled-out your athletic profile (using the forms found in the back of the book) describing your athletic achievements as well as academic achievements. As a family, you are going to get the home team (the athlete and his or her parents) practicing your approach for the successful interview. This manual, a vital and important guide, gives the home team a game plan to use before any college coach contacts you.

Pursuing an athletic scholarship is exactly like interviewing for a job. Even though you have skills, you have to convince the coach that you can add to his or her present program and be a positive addition to the university. The athlete and all of the members of the home team need to be well-prepared for the work that is to be done. The professional staff at the Mental Game Plan has had many years of experience training athletes in motivation, mental focusing, and scholarship search programs. You and your family will benefit from this program by following the suggestions in this manual.

Looking for a scholarship is a year-round job. There is no special time to contact the coach. Recruiting is an ongoing process! NCAA rules outline the time that a coach can contact you, but there are no restrictions on you contacting the coach. This is why you should have a plan to market yourself to all potential schools that offer scholarships starting in your junior year of high school. Remember, you only need to find one school that will offer you financial aid to pay for your education by offering your athletic skills in exchange for a college education.

Introduction

This manual is organized into four sections: the scholarship process, interview preparation, questions the coach might ask, and questions the athlete should ask. After both the family and athlete read this manual, practice the answers while at dinner between yourselves. Listen to the input and sharpen up your answers to the listed questions. Check out, review, and practice all the information that is in this booklet. Then get out and have fun competing for that available scholarship money. Don't be discouraged when you start. Twenty-three publishers rejected Dr. Seuss' first children's book. The twenty-fourth publisher sold six million copies of the book.

Section 1

The Scholarship Process

Billions of dollars in scholarship money goes unused each year because the student does not know how to apply for it. Over 70 percent of the colleges do not have adequate funds to actively recruit athletes with Division III and the NAIA hurt the most. Most college coaches rely on recommendations, profiles, game films, and personal contacts to select the college athlete. Over 350 colleges meet 100 percent of the financial needs of all college freshmen who qualify for need. Over nine hundred colleges give financial aid to 100 percent of all athletes who qualify. These are a mix of grants, loans, aid, and scholarships. Over 180 colleges give freshman over $7,000.

Only NCAA Division I and II give athletic scholarships. All others give financial aid, which is usually in the combined form of grants (that is, no repayment required), loans, and jobs. The coach is only

Kenneth Parady

allowed to personally meet the athlete twice. All colleges are under pressure by Title 9 to recruit and fund all women's sports teams at the same level as the men's programs. The women's recruiting system is far less effective than the men's, and most coaches rely upon word of mouth to recruit.

Section 2

Interview Preparation

Sell Yourself by Projecting Optimism

Concentrate on what you can do, not what you think you can do. Remember all of the positive things listed in your Mental Game Plan evaluation.[1] Review the athletic statistics on your profile. Let the coach know that you can help the team win and, in doing so, bring positive exposure to the coach, the college, and the team. Demonstrate confidence, interest, and enthusiasm.

Show in words that you can work for, with, and on a team. The coach is looking for team players. Stress that you are a team player. Use the Mental Game Plan evaluation on your profile to support your

---

[1] A variety of athletes from professional to high school for measurement of athletic mental characteristics use the Mental Game Plan evaluation. It is available through National Sports Marketing Group.

own personal athletic mental characteristics, such as competitiveness, commitment, mental toughness, and confidence.

The Recruiting Process

In their hands, college coaches should have a complete professional profile of your athletic and academic career and a photo. Interested colleges will respond to the athlete by phone or mail or have the administration office send out an application.

If you receive an application, fill it out and send it back to the coach immediately. If you delay, you may be removed from the school's recruiting process. Always return any correspondence directly to the coach.

The athlete must respond to all contacts even if there is no desire to attend this college. Keep a dated record of the contact and if it were by phone, letter, or in person. Your negotiations for a better offer down the road may depend on how many offers you have received in the past.

Personalized stationary (6 1/2" x 9 1/2") is recommended, and it should be used to reply to all contacts and requests for school literature. Use a felt tip pen, make it short, and always stress your interest in the college, the team, and the coach.

If a coach is serious about you, there will be a second meeting with him or her, a recruiter, athletic director, or possibly an alumnus. Remember, they will discuss you in detail at a private meeting later on, so sell yourself to everyone. One may be a mentor in the future. All interviews are considered for evaluation by the coach, so respond to all personnel you talked to, thanking them for their time, input, and consideration. You never know who will push your case in these review meetings.

After the coach's contact, start communicating with him or her, and reinforce your interest in his or her program. Don't bug him or her, but do correspond with him or her with any new information about you. Request more information about the college and your chances of playing for him or her. Be aggressive. After all, isn't that what he or she is looking for in an athlete? Be newsy and informative. Don't be overbearing.

By keeping a list of the names and addresses of the schools where your profile was sent, you can target the college that didn't respond to your profile. If you are interested in that school, write the coach! Send a copy of your profile, and ask if you could talk to him or her about the possibility of playing for his or her school. Informal meetings may be set up directly between the athlete and the coach. If possible, try to arrange a joint meeting with your high school coach at the school or your home. You will feel more comfortable when supporters surround you.

If the coach is serious about you, there will be a second meeting at the college. This is called a recruiting visit. You will meet other athletes and coaches. Remember, they will all discuss your behavior at a private meeting after you leave, so sell yourself to each person you meet. Any of these individuals may tip the interview in your favor and get you that position on the team.

Most importantly, never drink or party with the athletes you meet on this visit. After one bad move, you will lose everything you have worked so hard to achieve. Excuse yourself and retire early. Say you're tired.

Interviews are reviewed and discussed, so write all personnel you have talked to, thanking them for their input and consideration. You never know who will push your case in these review meetings.

When the best athlete is picked, the process of working out a financial aid package begins to be discussed. This process will involve negotiation, and the athlete should always counter the coach's offer for a better deal.

Dress Appropriately

Select an outfit and apparel that is neat and conservative. Shine your shoes, and have your outfit pressed.

Males

Select a white shirt and conservative tie (small figures, stripes, or soft colors). Choose a neat, well-fitting sports jacket and slacks or a navy blue, black, or gray suit. Wear dark, not white, socks and dark dress shoes, not tennis or athletic shoes.

Females

Select a conservative, not flashy, solid-colored dress with a jacket. Choose a solid-colored jacket and skirt with a solid-colored, conservative blouse. Wear closed, low- to mid-heel pumps and standard pantyhose, not textured or figured. Do not wear socks, pants, jeans, or tennis or athletic shoes. Avoid any fad clothing.

General Grooming

Males

Get a haircut or trim hair one week prior to the interview. Avoid weird haircuts because the coach isn't looking for a rock star. Be clean-shaven. Remove all earrings and jewelry.

Females

Wear your hair in a neat, conservative style. Leave fancy barrettes, hair accessories, and so forth at home. Wear only a minimum amount of makeup; wearing less is better.

General Appearance Tips

Keep all jewelry, bracelets, chains, and metals to a minimum. Look clean by attending to all the aspects of good personal grooming. Practice wearing your outfit to church so you will feel comfortable in it when you have to interview the coach.

Keep in mind that you get only one chance to make a good, positive first impression. Make it count!

Personal Issues

Coaches are not interested in your personal problems—significant others, cars, parents, teachers, curfews, or anything else you believe is a problem—so they are best left unmentioned. If anything is considered serious, inform the coach on how you have overcome it and how it will not become a problem. Honesty pays, and it will impress the coach.

Stay on track and only talk about two things: (1) your ability to play collegiate sports and (2) school, sports questions, and academic and career goals.

Listen and Observe

Answer any questions that the coach asks. Target your responses to the questions, and answer only what the coach asks you. Don't volunteer any unsolicited answers to questions not asked.

Listen to how the coach reacts to your answers and reply positively. Be aware during the interview of these reactions from a coach: strong interest, agreement, confusion, and boredom. These indicate how the interview is going. React to each individual reaction appropriately:

- **Strong Interest:** Be calm, handle the questions, and let the coach stay in charge. Respond with your own strong interest in the school. If you both have strong interest, close! Ask the coach if he or she has an interest in you because you have one in him or her.

- **Agreement:** Close the interview with "I like what I hear. Could I get back to you after I think about it?" Never say, "I will discuss this with my parents." You want to show that you are in control and mature and it will be your decision.
- **Confusion:** Ask questions so you can get back on stream. What is confusing the coach? You may have thrown him or her off by not seeming to be interested in his or her program. He or she may think you prefer another school. Make every coach think you want to play for him or her.
- **Boredom:** This is the worst type, and you may be wasting your time at this school. It would be better, if this continues, to confront the coach. Ask him or her if he or she is interested in you. Tell him or her you sense that he or she isn't. It may be better to terminate the interview. Always thank him or her for his time and leave on an upbeat note. He or she may talk to other coaches about you.

After the Interview

Write a brief note to the coach, thanking him or her for the opportunity to be interviewed, and state a strong interest in his or her athletic program. Review the interview in your mind and what you need to improve. Discuss all the interviews with the home team.

Rehearse your interviewing skills with the home team. Like in competitive sports, after losing, be up for your next interview.

Remember that you only need one offer for your scholarship/aid.

Section 3

Questions a Coach Might Ask

What Coaches Look for in the Interview

- Indications of character, drive, competence, and coach-ability
- Social and academic potential, along with conversational and sensibility skills
- An athlete who will make the coach look good and be a team player
- An athlete who will make his or her team a winner and promote the college's reputation
- Athletes who are coachable, will fit into the program, and get along well with other teammates and classmates

Most of all, the coach wants someone who he or she can relate to and who is receptive to coaching and continues to improve each year.

Standard Questions

- Why do you want to attend our school?
    - Give a clear, honest answer, and be informed about the college. State what abilities and skills you are able to bring to the school. Show an interest in academics and your desire to graduate. Mention that you want to work with a quality coach who can help you develop your talents and ability, on and off the practice field. Indicate that you can contribute to the athletic program at this school in academics as well as athletics.
    - Do not dwell on what the school can give. Instead, concentrate on what you can give to the school and its athletic and scholastic program. Stress dedication, achievement, determination, and your winning spirit in the classroom as well as on the field. Refer to your Mental Game Plan Evaluation for items to zero in on your abilities and attitudes that you can offer to a college.
- Which sports do you like best?
    - Stress your primary sport. Don't try to name a large number of sports. Coaches like to see that you are concentrated on one sport. Identify only the sports that you are proficient at on a competitive level. It shows that you are an all-around athlete, and it helps you in your main sport. Mention any awards, honors, and recognition you have received. Try to work it into

your conversation with the coach. Don't just rattle them off. The coach has your profile, and he or she can read.
- If you have an offseason training program, discuss in detail the program, its results, and benefits you have received from training.
- What are your long- and short-range goals?
  - This is an important question. Your answer will show that you are mature and have goals. Coaches like to see personal direction. Before the interview, list your goals, such as graduation and the profession you expect to pursue in the future. Practice working them into your discussion, along with your athletic goals. Tell the coach how the Mental Game Plan will improve your goal-setting skills. Explain how you are learning to focus and set objectives that will improve your athletic and personal goals. Colleges want dedication and a student who has focus. Only 47 percent of freshmen become sophomores. *Time* magazine's first employee stayed with the magazine for fifty-six years. That is dedication!
- What kind of college interests you?
  - This answer indicates your suitability for this college. If you are not interested in this school, do not waste your time. If you are interested, discuss the size, location, athletic, and academic reputation that you desire in a school. Ask questions.

- What are your strong and weak points?
  - The ability to talk about your strengths indicates your self-confidence. This discussion is your opportunity to talk about your achievements as presented in your profile.
  - As for your weaknesses, it is accurate to say, "None have been called to my attention that would prevent me from doing a good job for you in your program." We all have a few weak points. Tell the coach you are working to improve them. Ask if the coach feels comfortable about helping you overcome any you may have and what kind of program he or she has to help athletes develop their full potential. Do not put yourself down or continue to harp on your weak points. Talk about your positives from the coach's viewpoint. Never hide any weak points. Just don't volunteer them. Wait for the coach to ask. If it never comes up, it probably isn't important.
- What are your hobbies?
  - This is a "fishing expedition" question in several ways. It tells the coach about your outlook and attitudes. It is surprising how many tennis, golf, or single-player athletes have other solitary hobbies. If you are a singles athlete, let the coach know you have group interests. Strengthen your answer by pointing out these interests.

How to Interview the Coach

- Team athletes tend to have more gregarious interests. They enjoy meeting people, and it shows at school and during off-school activities. Talk about your community involvement, clubs, and so forth.
- What are your parents' occupations?
    - The coach is looking for your personal attitude in answering this question. Your answer will give clues to your personality. Are you defensive or confident? Do you feel your fate is doomed because your parents do not have a college education? Do you deride them for ethnic or religious interests? Do you alibi? Be proud of them! You are where you are because of your family, parents, or a role model. State that fact with confidence.
    - In your parents' time, anyone who graduated from high school was considered a success. For your information, Edwin Land dropped out of Harvard in his first year and invented the Polaroid camera.
- What are you looking for in a scholarship?
    - Do not ask for any dollar commitment from the coach. Let him or her tell you what he or she has to offer. The coach knows what is available for your sport. He or she also is aware of other funds and pools of monies available within the department. If you mention a dollar figure like, "Coach, I was hoping for a fifteen thousand-dollar scholarship" and

find out the coach had twenty to thirty thousand funded for a scholarship, you have just lost five to ten thousand dollars. Do not ask for specific numbers in financial aid! Let the coach make the offer. Ask the coach what funds are available for an athlete with your skills and if you have to repay the grants. And if so, when?

- If your grades, SAT, or ACT are good, ask the coach to help you obtain some academic aid to match his or her athletic money so you can play for him or her. If you perform well in your first year, he or she can give you a full ride in your second because you would have earned it.

- Help the coach figure out a way to recruit you. It is up to him or her to handle the details. He or she only needs direction. Most athletes don't come with a high academic résumé. Let him or her know you have one.

- When asked if your parents can afford to help pay for your education, say no. Don't discuss your parents' family income. You don't know anything about it. State what you want in order to make it on your own, a full ride! Show that you plan to finance your own education through your academic and athletic abilities. Remember, all you need is the coach's help to get that aid.

***

The following questions have no standard answers but should be discussed with your home team for an appropriate answer that fits the athlete. Try to answer positively by mentally rehearsing how you would answer these questions if brought up in a coach's interview.

- Why do you want to play on our team?
  - Be honest and positive, and state your need for a coach that can give you a program for improvement in both academics and athletics.
- How do you rate yourself as a player?
  - Use your past high school athletic history, and project the same attitude that got you through your high school experience. Be realistic. Evaluate your size, speed, desire, and the people who are going to be your competitors. Be confident in your evaluation.
- What other colleges are looking at you?
  - This is the reason you do not turn down any offers with colleges that contact you. These offers may get you a better offer. In most cases, colleges trust each other and use that as a competitive reference.
  - Let the coach know you have taken the Mental Game Plan[2] by Dr. Thomas Tutko, San Jose State University, and have an athletic profile workbook you are using to improve your

---

[2] See order form in the back of the book.

athletic attitude. These results and workbook program will help him understand how to communicate with you and will define your attitudes.

- Tell the coach that you have several schools looking at you but are not at liberty to discuss them. As you receive contacts from various colleges, you will attain a core list of schools that you can use to discuss with future college contacts.

- What motivates you?
  - Don't be egotistical. Stay away from the "I" factor. Family, friends, education, and the desire to contribute to society should motivate you. Remember, you are a team player.

- What are your three most important accomplishments?
  - Discuss this question with the home team. Evaluate your high school career, both athletic and academic, for example, community service, academic achievement, making the school team, and so forth.

- Could you give an example of your athletic attitude?
  - These characteristics are listed in your mental evaluation. Combine the strong points of each one, and try to make a short statement of your mental attitudes. Use a combination of these strengths to make a positive statement.
  - The Mental Game Plan evaluation matches your attitudes with other athletes on a national basis. The results give you validity

of your strengths against over a half-million other athletes. Dr. Thomas Tutko developed this program for the evaluation of professional and Olympian athletes, and most major league teams in all sports use it.

- Could you give an example of some of your leadership skills?
    - Point out objective things in your life that would show your leadership skills. Use examples such as class offices, team captain, community recognition, political activities, and so forth.
- How have you helped former teams win?
    - Describe decisive plays that helped you win a contest. Go back to Little League, recreation ball, high school, summer camps, and so forth. Summarize the statement by describing your one characteristic that helped your team win these games.
- Do you consider yourself a competitive person? Explain.
    - Use examples in athletics, academics, family, community, and so forth. The reason you are competitive should be the same for all forms of activities.
- Why do you feel you have college potential?
    - Base your statement on past successes and not future potential. Use experiences from high school, recreation, work experience, sports, character, religious, community, and so forth.
- How did you get along with your coaches?

- Tell the truth. Be positive. If you have had a negative experience, explain that you tried hard to do what the coach wanted but you just didn't work well together. Stress that you learned a lot from this experience and you are much better prepared to understand your future coaches' demands. It was a hard but great learning experience. We can't get along with everyone, but if we learn to accept the results, we can improve. No one expects for everyone to love you. An athlete that always denies that it's his or her fault is suspect.

- In the Roman Empire's first year, one of the founders killed the other founder (his brother) over a land dispute. Disagreement has been with us for over five thousand years. You must learn from it and move on with your life.

- Why do you want to go to this college?
    - You should have received your college literature before you talk to the coach. Read about the college and use that information as your basis for wanting to attend this school. Be informed. If you have relatives or friends that attended this college, bring this up. There are priorities for family graduates. Friends also help.

- What will be your biggest contribution to this team?
    - Focus on you being a team player. Let the coach know that, if you play, you can help him or her win. If you don't play, he or she can count on you to work extra hard to push the starting players, but you expect to start based on your performance. Let the coach know that, if you don't start, you will work extra hard for him. You have the work ethic to succeed and only need a chance.
- What kind of team members do you like best?
    - Be open-minded on this question. Don't box yourself into defining the type of players you want to be around. Remember, the team may change each year. Tell the coach that you like people who "want to win" and you can play with all kinds of athletes.
- What kind of players annoys you?
    - Answer the following: players who give up, players who are not team players, players who don't put out 100 percent, and so forth. Even though these players may annoy you, your positive attitude can help motivate these players if you are part of the team.

- What are your feelings about drug testing?
  - Don't hesitate! State that you don't do drugs and you feel drug testing is necessary to keep the cheaters out of college athletics.
- How would you describe the "ideal coach"?
  - Think back to your favorite coach, and make a list of his strong characteristics. Use this list to compose a statement about what you consider is your ideal coach. You can't go wrong with the statement that you really are looking for leadership in a coach. Be general. Don't describe a saint. You may want a quiet, low-key coach, and the person you are talking to is a raving maniac on the field. Let him or her know that you can play for any coach who has an underlying concern for the interests of his or her players and who you can look up to in directing you throughout your sports career. Show more concern about what you can learn from your college coach. State that you want a college experience that you can take with you into life after graduation.

***

The questions you ask regarding the college, its academic program, and its athletic department tell as much about your attitude as the answers you give to the coach's questions. By asking the right questions, you underline your desire to understand the coach's expectations and to be reasonably sure you will find the right college that will challenge you.

The objective is to be as well informed as possible about the college and its programs before making a school choice. Do not take the coaches interview lightly.

Section 4

Questions an Athlete Should Ask

- What are the practice responsibilities of the athletes?
    - Don't ask this question in a negative way. Let the coach know you want to get the rules so you may understand what you have to do to succeed with this team. Stress to the coach that you think practice is as important to a team's success as the actual game. Ask if he or she has an offseason training program for his players? Is this coaching program designed to help you improve as an athlete through working in this training program?
- How about your teammates?
    - Ask who would be your teammates and from what areas. How many seniors are returning? How many lettermen? How many freshmen? Do many freshmen play? Do the athletes room

together and so forth? How many freshmen and sophomores have started for the team in the past five or six years? How many have played all four years?

- What is the school's athletic and academic standing?
  - What percentage of athletes graduates from the school? Do they graduate in four years? Is your sport financially stable? Are tutors available for the athlete? Does the coaching staff support the athlete in the classroom?
  - How tough is the athletic schedule? How much classwork is missed because of team travel and out-of-state overnight games?
  - Where does the team stand in the country in its athletic program? How is its academic program regarded throughout the country?
- How have athletes who have a background like mine succeed?
  - Did they graduate, drop out of school, or take four or five years to graduate? How many continued on for a post-graduate degree? Did they have any trouble handling the schoolwork, and did they use any academic advisors? What is the GPA average of the team? May I contact some former athletes and talk to them?

- What are the coach's responsibilities to the athlete?
  - What does the coach personally look for in recruiting an athlete? How many credits do I need each term/quarter to keep my scholarship/aid? Does the aid package include summer school? What happens to my scholarship/aid if I get injured playing for this school? What happens to my aid if I am injured during the offseason? If I don't make the team as a freshman, will you redshirt me? How much help will I receive in transferring to another school if I lose my scholarship/aid through no fault of my own, such as discontinuation of the sport? What GPA do I need to continue playing for the team? Will I receive a written contract of my scholarship/aid? Will my scholarship/aid be for four or five years?

***

These questions will help you make a solid decision as to whether you want to attend this school or not. Ask them in a nonthreatening but informative way. Never act arrogant or aloof. You are attempting to match your qualities with the school's qualities so you both benefit. Remember, you will have a long-term relationship with this school. Make sure you both want each other.

If you receive an offer of interest but do not wish to attend that college, write a thank-you note to the coach. Athletics has a unique bonding between individuals. Each coach respects the other coaches' opinions. He or she may recommend you to another coach. If you have a good interview with a coach who can't give you a scholarship, ask him or her to recommend you to another school that he or she thinks may have an interest. This is called networking, and it works.

Good luck and go get 'em!

NATIONAL SPORTS MARKETING GROUP

LETTERS OF INTENT

All NCAA Division I conferences in the letter of intent program recognize each other's agreements and consider them binding. The only Division I conference that does not recognize the letter of intent, is the Ivy League, which offers aid but no athletic scholarships.

The letter is a binding contract between the athlete and the institution. Once an institution offers a scholarship with the letter and it is signed by the athlete and his or her legal guardians, the athlete has committed to attend that institution for one full academic year. A scholarship must be offered for the letter to be valid.

There are ways to declare the letter of intent void:

* If the student is not admitted to the institution or does not meet the academic eligibility requirements.

* Through mutual agreement of the athletic director and student.

* By not attending any institution honoring the letters of intent for one full academic year (for example, enrollment in junior college).

* Service in the US armed forces or on a church mission for at least 18 months.

* If the sport has been discontinued at the institution.

* If the institution has violated NCAA or conference regulations in the recruiting of the athlete.

Athletes are only allowed to sign one letter of intent and the violation of the agreement carries a stiff penalty. If an athlete does not attend the institution for one full academic year and enrolls in another school with the letter of intent program, the athlete cannot compete for two full academic years and loses two years of eligibility in athletics.

NATIONAL SPORTS MARKETING GROUP

THE ATHLETE WORKBOOK

HOW TO USE THIS WOOKBOOK

This binder will make it easy for you to gather all the information necessary to prepare your ATHLETIC INTRODUCTION for your scholarship marketing campaign. Fill out each and every question to the best of your ability. If you do not have an answer, please place a slash in the space. The more information you gather, the better your profile will look to the college coach.

Documents contained in this book included:

The Student Application

Parent/Athlete information

Mental Game Plan test

College Division selection

Photo selection & specifications

Reference forms to give out

- (1) Grade Transcript to school office. SAT/ACT/GPA & Class Rank.
- (2) Coaches Athletic evaluations.
- (1) Teacher Evaluation, core subject. English, Math, Science, etc.

THE WORKBOOK

Keeping the Workbook bound and intact, sign the Contract, complete the Mental Game Plan and fill out all questions in the Parent/Athlete Evaluation, Athlete Division Evaluation and enclose (2) 3" x 4" Action Photographs, Black & White or Color with a **light** background. A **CLOSE UP** view (knees up) of the athlete is the best photo.

Return the workbook to the address listed below and a copy of the signed contract will be returned to you. Your data will be kept confidential and will be used to prepare your personal athletic introduction and Mental Game Plan.

In the meantime, forms marked "Coach's, Teachers Evaluation and Transcript Release" are to be given to two (2) coaches, a (1) core subject teacher and your school administrative office. Instruct them to fill out the Transcript form **as soon as possible** and mail it to NSMG.

STUDENT APLICATION FORM
(Please print)

Date _____

PERSONAL

Name _____
Address _____
City _____ State _____ Zip _____
Yr/graduation _____ Birthday _____ Birthplace _____

FAMILY

Parent(s) Name Mother _____ Father _____
Home Phone ( ) _____ Bus ( ) _____ Fax ( ) _____
email _____

Occupation /Mother _____ Father _____
Education/Mother _____ Father _____

Family athletic history
_____
_____
_____

ACCADEMICS

High School _____ Size _____
Address _____
City _____ State ____ Zip ____ Phone ( ) ____
Times on Honor Roll _____ College Major _____
School size ____ Class Rank ____ GPA ____ SAT ____ ACT ____

STRONGEST SUBJECTS

Languages taken

_____
_____
_____

Math	____	Science	____
Art	____	Computors	____
English	____	History	____
Gov't	____	Psychology	____
Pub Speak	____	Literature	____
Debate	____	Drama	____
Acctg	____	Electronics	____
Algebra	____	Chemistry	____
Physics	____	Economics	____

NATIONAL SPORTS MARKETING GROUP

Student Appliction, Page 2

Advance Placement Courses taken _____

Special talents or hobbies _____

Activities you participate in outside of school _____

School Clubs, Organizations and offices held _____

Community involvement, volunteer work, part time jobs _____

Sex ____ Religion _____ Ra ce _____ Nationality _____

Do you plan to obtain a graduate degree? _____ Any health problems? _____

Explain _____

Do you think you can handle college life? Tel l me Why.

NATIONAL SPORTS MARKETING GROUP

ATHLETIC EVALUATION
PARENT/ATHLETE
(PLEASE PRINT)

NAME _____

FIRST SPORT _____
Position (1) _____ Height _____
Position (2) _____ Weight _____
Coaches name _____ Chest _____
                                                   Waist _____
* SECOND SPORT _____ Neck _____
Position (1) _____ Vertical
Position (2) _____ Jump _____
Coaches name _____

Total letters won _____ 1st sport _____ 2nd sport _____ 3rd sport _____
Speed (40 yd) _____ Other speed _____ Weight/Lift-Squat _____ Bench Press _____
Other times _____

FIRST SPORT - ATHLETIC ACHIEVEMENTS

ATHLETIC HONORS
Athletic awards _____
Recognition in - League _____ County _____ State _____
Other Recognition _____

TEAM RECOGNITON
Team honors (Scoring, Hits, Assists, etc) _____
Individual honors (Captain, MVP, etc.) _____

Camp/outside awards _____ Tournament awards _____
Years played sport _____ Years as starter _____ Rank on team _____
Athletic records School _____ League _____ State _____

OUTSIDE SPORTS PROGRAMS

CAMPS, LEAGUES, SPORTS TOURNAMENTS, CLUBS ATTENDED, ETC.

_____
_____
_____

NATIONAL SPORTS MARKETING GROUP

Ath Evaluation, Page 2

Description of Athlete FIRST SPORT (Use words from attached chart)
_____
_____
_____
_____

* SECOND SPORT - ATHLETIC ACHIEVEMENTS

Athletic Honors _____
Individual honors (Captain, MVP, ect.) _____
Years Played Sport_____ Years As Starter _____ Rank on Team _____

TEAM/LEAGUE HONORS
Team _____ League _____ County _____
Camp/Outside _____
Other recognition _____

CAMPS, OUTSIDE LEAGUES, SPORTS TOURNAMENTS, etc. (Awards, Honors)
_____
_____
_____

Second sport
 Descripton of Athlete (Use words from attached chart)
_____
_____
_____
_____

Why do you think you can play college ball, and what can you contribute to the team?
_____
_____
_____
_____

NATIONAL SPORTS MARKETING GROUP

COACHES EVALUATION

Date _____

Athletes Name _____
Coaches Name _____ Phone _____
School _____
Athletes ratings   Time/40 _____ Vertical Jump _____ Press _____ Lift/Squat _____
Hiting, scoring average per game, etc. _____
Other ratings _____
Athlete's Sport _____ Position (s) 1st _____ 2nd _____
School League _____ Won/Loss Record _____
School Rating in the State: _____ County _____ League _____

(Use words on next page to help describe the athlete)

ATHLETIC SKILLS/ACHIEVEMENTS: List any team, league, personal awards, records, etc.

_____
_____
_____
_____
_____

PHYSICAL DESCRIPTIONS: Describe physical, mental strengths and skills, etc.

_____
_____
_____
_____
_____

COLLEGE POTENTIAL: When could this athlete start in college, potential in college, etc.

_____
_____
_____
_____

COACH, TELL ME! What has this athlete contributed to the team, school and you personally.

_____
_____
_____
_____
_____

Please complete & return to athete promptly.

NATIONAL SPORTS MARKETING GROUP

COACHES EVALUATION

Date _____

Athletes Name _____
Coaches Name _____ Phone _____
School _____
Athletes ratings Time/40 _____ Vertical Jump _____ Press _____ Lift/Squat _____
Hiting, scoring average per game, etc. _____
Other ratings _____
Athlete's Sport _____ Position (s) 1st _____ 2nd _____
School League _____ Won/Loss Record _____
School Rating in the State: _____ County _____ League _____

(Use words on next page to help describe the athlete)

ATHLETIC SKILLS/ACHIEVEMENTS: List any team, league, personal awards, records, etc.

_____
_____
_____
_____

PHYSICAL DESCRIPTIONS: Describe physical, mental strengths and skills, etc.

_____
_____
_____
_____

COLLEGE POTENTIAL: When could this athlete start in college, potential in college, etc.

_____
_____
_____
_____

COACH, TELL ME! What has this athlete contributed to the team, school and you personally.

_____
_____
_____
_____

Please complete & return to athete promptly.

NATIONAL SPORTS MARKETING GROUP

TEACHERS EVALUATION

Student Name: _____ Date: _____
Teacher: _____ Subject: _____
School: _____ Phone: _____
Student Academic Honors: _____

The above student has given you this form for completion. The contents will be used to profile this student for a potential athletic scholarship. We know your time is valuable and your effort on behalf of this student is "greatly" appreciated.

Please comment on the following areas:

Academic Skills; Quality of work; Level of achievement

Homework performance; Organization of work; Pride in work

Individual/Group participation; Respect for authority and Leadership

Areas of accomplishments; Advanced level of work

In what school functions, organizations, etc. does this student participate?

NATIONAL SPORTS MARKETING GROUP
Teachers Evaluation
Page 2

Attitudes and Habits: Describe this students' teachability, character, mental attitude, determination, goal setting skills, personal drive, special talent, etc.

_____
_____
_____
_____

College Potential: Academic capabilities, self motivation, desire and maturity.

_____
_____
_____
_____

Check each of the following items which apply to the student:

_____	Quick learner	_____	Is a classroom leader
_____	Seen as a leader by others	_____	Is liked by others
_____	Has pride in classwork	_____	Gets work done on time
_____	Work is done ahead of time	_____	Can balance academics/athletics
_____	Interfaces with teachers	_____	Serious about education

How will this student function while adjusting to the first year of college?

_____
_____
_____
_____
_____

Please complete & return promptly to student.

NATIONAL SPORTS MARKETING GROUP

ATHLETE DIVISION EVALUTION

Athlete Name _____ Sport _____

School _____ Postion _____

Coach _____ Phone _____

	Coach	NSMG	Athlete/Parent	Min. GPA
TOP 75 Colleges	___	___	___	2.0
DIV 1A	___	___	___	2.0
DIV 1AA	___	___	___	2.0
DIV II	___	___	___	2.0
DIV III	___	___	___	2.5
NAIA	___	___	___	2.5
IVY LEAGUE	___	___	___	3.5
MILITARY	___	___	___	3.0

Coach: Please check the appropriate divisions that you believe this athlete could complete
Athlete: Check all divisions where you think you could compete. Be sure to observe the listed requirements below and the GPA required.

Div 1 TOP PLAYER IN STATE, physical, All-State, All-Conference, 3 year starter.

Div 2 TOP PLAYER IN AREA, 2 year starter, standout in conference, all area, MVP.

Div 3 SCHOOL STANDOUT, 2 year starter, good GPA, high college academic potential.

NAIA STARTER, good GPA, good mental attitude, character, good athlete.

Military TOP ACADEMIC, wants military, excellent athlete, top moral character.

Ivy League: Excels in academics, high SAT/ACT (1300 SAT+) good academic GPA, (3.5).

Do not write in this space - for NSMG reference

DIV 1 _____ DIV 2 _____ DIV 3 _____ NACA _____ IVY _____

STATES (3) _____ _____ _____

REGIONS   NO _____ SO _____ EAST _____ WEST _____ .

ATHLETIC INTRODUCTION

2/21/97

SAMPLE ATHLETE

7 Smith Street
Orange County   CA 92679

Year/Grad:	1994
Sport:	Volleyball
Position:	Outside Hitter
Coach:	Bob Smith
High School:	Highlands High School
	300 Bridge Street
	Orange County, CA 92688
H.S. Phone:	(800) 555-5555

B/D: 01/07/76 **Neck:** 0 **Bench Press:** 85 lbs
Height: 5'8" **Chest:** 0 **Lift/ Squat:** 95 lbs
Weight: 130lbs. **Waist:** 0 **Vertical Jump:** 26"
Other Times/ Strengths: **Speed:** 0

League: Seaview
Advisor: Jim Olsen
Parent: Mr Mrs Athlete
Home Phone: (800) 555-5555

Holds The Position Over Older Players Because Of Her Excellent Speed, Movement & Good Reaction To The Ball; Gets M From Her Natural Ability & Arm Swing Which Allows Her To Make Great Kills; Great Blocker; Is Fast Defensively; Gets To Hard Balls Easily; Great Attitude For Coaching; Excellent Work Ethic; Never Misses Practice And Works Hard While She Is There; Constantly Strives To Be Better; Accepts Coaching Suggestions Easily; Pushes Herself With Little Coaching; Possesses A Strong Frame And Will Gain Strength Over The Next Two Years; Excellent Vertical Jump Around The Net; Adjust Quickly To Game Circumstances; Excellent Form; Playing Club Volleyball In The Most Competitive Volleyball Area In The Country.

Team Honors:
Team Blocking Leader; Varsity Basketball Most Inspirational Player; Most Valuable Runner; Most Valuable Player In Basketball; Recognized As Team Leader As A Sophomore; Assists Leader, Basketball; Steal Leader; Captain; 3 Year Starter.

Varsity Letters: Four Letter Winner

League Honors:
All Tournament Team, Basketball; All League, Honorable Mention; Played On A Team With A 60-30 Record In Tough League; Team Placed Third In League In '91; All League In Basketball; Started On Varsity Basketball Team In Sophomore Year.

Other Sports:
Strong Three Sport Star; Excellent Basketball Player; Played In Mission Viejo Vollyball Club League For Past Two Years; Recognize As Strong Tournament Player In Basketball League; Versatile Athlete; CSF (California Scholastic Federation)

CLASS
Size: 333
Rank: 104
GPA: 3.5
SAT: 995
ACT: 24

College Major: General Business

Academic Honors:
Senior Class President; Enviromental Club Involvement; CSF; Sports Commissioner; Referee At Grade Sch Volleyball Tournaments; Extremely Organized Student; Strong College Potential; Above Average Academic Skills, High Quality Of Work; Excellent Level Of Achievement; Strong Homework Performance; Has Pride in Her Work; Honors History Class; Performing Well In College History Program; Active In Junior Achievement Good Focus; Intelligent Student; Serious About Her Education; Comes From A Strong Academic Athletic Parents Are Involved.

NSMG Athletic Mental Appraisal:
A Competitive Person And Enjoys Challenges; Functions As Well As She Can And Is Disappointed If She Doesn't; Sets Achieveable Standards And Trys To Attain Them; Winning Is Important To Her; Is A Hard Worker; Does Not Bother Her To Put A Lot Of Extra Time To Be Successful; Never Quits Until She Perfects A Skill; Coaches Would Say She Is A Dedicated Player; An Assertive Person; Enjoys Taking Charge; Never Intimidated; Enjoys Being A Dominant Force; Has Faith In Her Ability; Is A To Concentrate Without Too Much Difficulty; Can Ignore Distraction And Annoyances With Minimal Problems; Has Great Cont Over Her Feelings; Her Ability To Make Decisions In An Emotional Part Of The Game Is Outstanding; Functions Like A Machin Great Under Pressure; Enjoys Pressure Situations; Great Ability Controlling Pressure When It Occurs.

2/21/15

Athletic Introduction

Sample Athlete

7 Smith Street

Orange County, CA 92679

B/D: 01/07/97

Height: 5'8"

Weight: 130 lbs.

Neck: 0

Chest: 0

Waist: 0

Other Times/Strengths:

    Bench Press: 85 lbs.

    Lift/ Squat: 95 lbs.

    Vertical Jump: 26"

    Speed: 0

Year Grad: 1994

Sport: Volleyball

Position: Outside Hitter

Coach: Bob Smith

High School: Highlands High School, 300 Bridge Street, Orange County, CA 92688

HS Phone: (800) 555-5555

League: Seaview

Advisor: Jim Olsen

Parent: Mr. and Mrs. Athlete

Home Phone: (800) 555-5555

- Holds the position over older players because of her excellent speed, movement, and good reaction to the ball
- Gets momentum from her natural ability and arm swing, which allows her to make great kills
- Is a great blocker
- Is fast defensively
- Gets to hard balls easily
- Has great attitude for coaching and excellent work ethic
- Never misses practice and works hard while she is there
- Constantly strives to be better
- Accepts coaching suggestions easily
- Pushes herself with little coaching
- Possesses a strong frame and will gain strength over the next two years
- Has excellent vertical jump around the net
- Adjusts quickly to game circumstances
- Has excellent form
- Plays club volleyball in the most competitive volleyball area in the country

Team Honors

- Team blocking leader
- Most Inspirational Player (varsity basketball)
- Most Valuable Runner
- MVP (basketball)
- Sophomore team leader
- Assists leader (basketball)
- Steal leader
- Captain
- Three-year starter

Varsity Letters

- Four-letter winner

League Honors

- All-Tournament Team (basketball)
- Honorable Mention (All League)
- Played on a team with a 60-30 record in tough league
- Team placed third in league in 1991
- All League (basketball)
- Started on varsity basketball team in sophomore year

Other Sports

- Strong three-sport star
- Excellent basketball player
- Played in Mission Viejo Volleyball Club League for past two years

- Recognized as strong tournament player in basketball league
- Versatile athlete
- CSF (California Scholastic Federation)

Class

Size: 333

Rank: 104

GPA: 3.5

SAT: 995

ACT: 24

College Major

- General business

Academic Honors

- Senior class president
- Environmental Club involvement
- CSF
- Sports commissioner
- Referee at grade school volleyball tournaments
- Extremely organized student
- Strong college potential
- Above average academic skills
- High quality of work
- Excellent level of achievement
- Strong homework performance

- Has pride in her work
- Honors history class
- Performs well in college history program
- Active in junior achievement
- Good focus
- Intelligent student
- Serious about her education
- Comes from a strong academic athlete
- Involved parents

NSMG Athletic Mental Appraisal

- A competitive person who enjoys challenges
- Functions as well as she can and is disappointed if she doesn't
- Sets achievable standards and tries to attain them
- Winning is important to her
- Is a hard worker
- Does not bother her to put a lot of extra time to be successful
- Never quits until she perfects a skill
- Coaches would say she is a dedicated player
- An assertive person
- Enjoys taking charge
- Never intimidated
- Enjoys being a dominant force
- Has faith in her ability

- Is able to concentrate without too much difficulty
- Can ignore distraction and annoyances with minimal problems
- Has great control over her feelings
- Her ability to make decisions in an emotional part of the game is outstanding
- Functions like a machine (great under pressure)
- Enjoys pressure situations
- Great ability controlling pressure when it occurs

NATIONAL SPORTS MARKETING GROUP

KEY ATHLETIC WORD LIST
(Words to help describe your athlete)

ATHLETIC SKILLS & ACHIEVEMENTS	PHYSICAL DESCRIPTIONS	COLLEGE POTENTIAL
QUICK	AGGRESSIVE	MULTIPLE SPORTS
LANKY	SOLID ATHLETE	IS ATTENTIVE
POWERFUL	DRIVEN	HAS HIGH HONORS
LONG ARMS	PASSIVE	HAS INTEGRITY
STRONG WRISTS	GOOD COMMUNICATOR	LETTER WINNER
SMOOTH SWING	AMBITIOUS	ACADEMIC STUDENT
HIGH KICK	HAS GROWTH GOALS	STATE AWARDS
A HITTER	IS SERIOUS	STRONG IN SPORTS
FAST	A LEADER	TOUGH LEAGUE
STRONG TACKLER	VARSITY PLAYER	DEDICATED
GREAT EYE	DEPENDABLE	STATE RANKED
GOOD TIMING	GOOD TRAINING	CIVIC INVOLVEMENT
GOOD HANDS	GOOD INSTINCTS	MOTIVATED
FORCES ACTION	DISCIPLINED	RESPECTED
A TEAM LEADER	IS DECISIVE	HAS CAREER GOALS
TOUGH	ADJUSTS QUICKLY	GOOD COUNTY RANK
PHYSICALLY STRONG	HANDLES PRESSURE	TOPS IN LEAGUE
GOOD SHOOTING EYE	STAYS COOL	WELL LIKED
GOOD BODY CONTROL	RESPONSIBLE	ALL TOURNAMENT
COACHABLE	IS COMPETITIVE	ALL CITY
GREAT BLOCKER	WANTS TO IMPROVE	SPORTS FAMILY
TEAM PLAYER	CONTROLLED	GOOD POTENTIAL
HAS SCORING ABILITY	GETS ALONG WITH PEERS	ALL STATE
GOOD FIELDING SKILLS	HAS CONFIDENCE	PLAYS OTHER SPORTS
A DECISION MAKER	DETERMINED	IS A CHRISTIAN
ALL COUNTY	SELF-CONFIDENT	WORKS YEAR AROUND
A RECORD SETTER	IS CONSCIENTIOUS	PLAYS ALL SPORTS
FLEXABLE	MAKES ADJUSTMENTS	CLOSE FAMILY
GOOD FORM	MENTALLY TOUGH	COMMUNITY LEADER
QUICK FEET	TAKES CHARGE	A LEADER
GOOD VERTICAL JUMP	HAS DESIRE	MOST IMPROVED PLAYER
A NATURAL TALENT	TIRELESS COMPETITOR	MOST VALUABLE
A SCRAMBLER	WANTS TO WIN	IS RESPONSIBLE
QUICK STARTER	PERSISTENT	TRUST WORTHY
A HUSTLER	HAS VERSATILITY	EMOTIONAL CONTROL

NATIONAL SPORTS MARKETING GROUP

YOUR "ACTION" PHOTOGRAPH

The photograph you submit for your ATHLETIC PROFILE should illustrate over-all body size, proportions and action/alertness.

Please gather TWO (2) action shots of you in your uniform. The picture should show YOU as the main person in the photo. College coaches will be looking at body size, leg/arm size, muscle structure and body strength. The size of the picture should be 3" x 5".

The photo should be as bright as possible, (shots in the daytime), dark shots will not reproduce well on your profile. A perfect shot of you is one that fills the picture from your knees to your head. No graduation photos.

These examples will help illustrate appropriate photos:

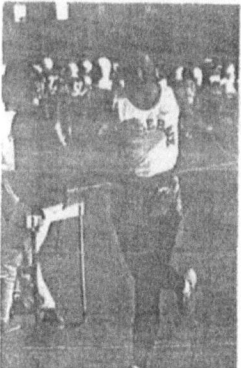
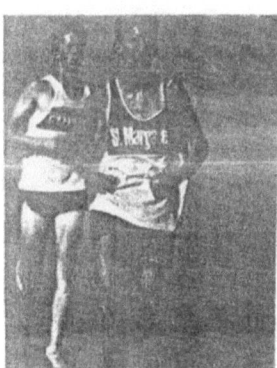
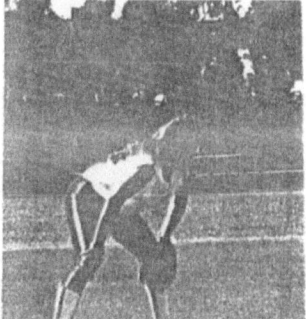
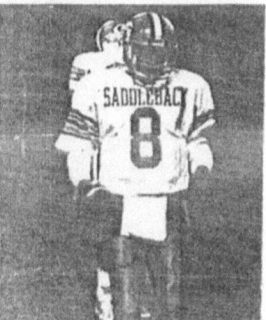

NATIONAL SPORTS MARKETING GROUP

NOTES

THE MENTAL GAME PLAN

"It's not the will to win that matters.... everyone has that.
It's the will to prepare to win that matters".
Paul "Bear" Bryant,
Football Coach, Alabama University

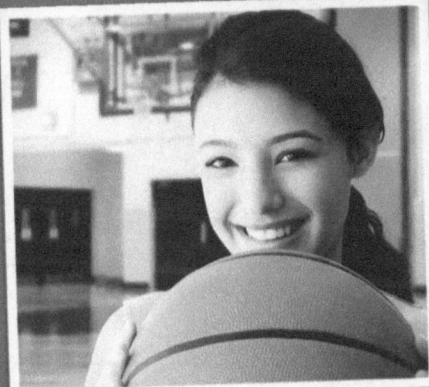

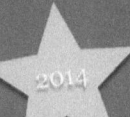

- Competitiveness
- Commitment
- Assertive
- Confidence
- Concentration
- Emotion Control
- Game Pressure

Men & Women Athletes

* Teaches goal setting skills.
* Improves game performance.
* Evaluates team mental attitudes.
* Sharpens player-coach communication.
* Enhances players performance.
* Forms co-operation between coach & parents.

Visit our Site to place orders, pricing & articles by coaches who used the MGP program.

http://www.mentalgame.com

The Mental Game Plan, 3027 Poplar Creek Dr. SE, #203, Kentwood, MI 49512-5665

Phone/Fax 616-827-0278, email: mentalgame@sbcglobal.net

THE MENTAL GAME PLAN
Athlete's Report

Name: Sample, Joe
School: Union High
Sport: Tennis
Date: October 2nd, 1996

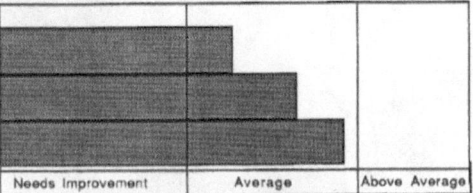

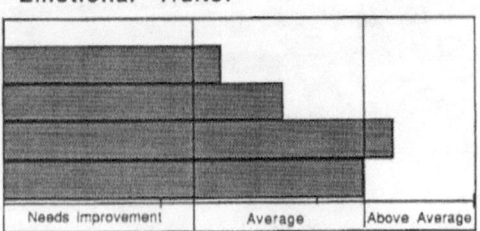

NOTE: If this test was taken honestly, it will not result in a negative report, but will help define your athletic mental attitudes against thousands of other athletes. If you implement this program, you will improve your mental skills which will help enhance your athletic performance. The results of this inventory should be shared with your coach and parents so they can help you in your mental development program.

* Copywrited © in 1989 by Kenneth T. Parady, NSMG

The Mental Game Plan

Athlete's Report

Name: Sample, Joe

School: Union High

Sport: Tennis

Date: October 2, 2014

Behavioral Traits

Emotional Traits

Note

If this test were taken honestly, it will not result in a negative report, but it will help define your athletic mental attitudes against thousands of other athletes. If you implement this program, you will improve your mental skills, which will help enhance your athletic performance. The results of this inventory should be shared with your coach and parents so they can help you in your mental development program.

Copyright © 1989 by Kenneth T. Parady, NSMG, and Dr. Thomas Tutko, San Jose State University

FINAL COLLEGE SELECTION CONTACT LIST

School Name	Contact	Letter	Phone/Pers

www.ingramcontent.com/pod-product-compliance
Lightning Source LLC
Chambersburg PA
CBHW021026180526
45163CB00005B/2129